I0435579

IT WORKS FOR ME

A Revolutionary Way of Eating

SANDRA RANDLES

3/1/2015

EDITED BY: SANDY HENDRICKSON

IT WORKS FOR ME
A Revolutionary Way of Eating

CreateSpace

Nutrition /diet

ISBN – 10: 1506114970
ISBN – 13: 978-1506114972

DEDICATION

To my husband, Don who walked beside me through all my diet challenges.

Since you have started your own Revolutionary Way of Eating, I wish you luck in your weight loss, as you discover that it will "Work For You" too!

Contents

Introduction   1

1. Giving up sweets   4

2. Giving up breads   13

3. Adding more fats   19

4. Protein and exercise   27

5. Today's diets   34

6. This is what works for me   42

INTRODUCTION

Every year is the same. It is New Year's Eve and I tell myself "Sandy, this is the year that you are going to take off this weight and keep it off." It is the same speech many of us give ourselves when we are making our New Year's resolutions. We make these resolutions with good intentions, but before long we find ourselves slipping back into the same old habits.

In the past when I tried to change the way I ate, I felt deprived and it seemed as if I was being punished for the weight I had gained. Because I overindulged, I had to suffer in order to lose the excess fat. Deprive myself, be hungry and pay the price. I have tried many different diets and would lose a few pounds only to have them gradually sneak back on. What was I doing wrong, why does it have to be such a struggle? There must be a painless way to lose weight and I am determined to find it.

I need to figure out my relationship with food. Why do I crave sweets? Why do I feel the need to snack? What are my comfort foods, the foods I turn to when I am feeling down or depressed? What put me on this cycle of overeating and eating the wrong foods and how do I change it?

Can overeating be an addiction? When you are addicted to cigarettes, you stop the habit by not

1

smoking. If eating is addictive, then how do you give up food? How do you stop the habit of overeating when it is a necessity to eat every day?

Is being overweight an inherited tendency or is it more complicated than that? Does obesity run in families or is it because family members may have the same habits of snacking, eating the wrong foods and overindulging.

Is overeating related more to habit or hunger? A baby will stop eating when he is feeling full. As adults, we sometimes eat just because it tastes good, even when we are full.

I don't know all the answers. I am not a nutritionist or an expert of any kind. I am just someone who has spent a large part of my adult life being overweight. I have tried many diets that have failed. I want to lose this weight forever.

The so called experts have given us advice for many decades with charts, pyramids, the do's and don'ts of healthy eating. Count calories, don't count calories, eat eggs, don't eat eggs, eating fats is ok eating fats is not ok. Americans are more overweight than they have ever been. Maybe the experts should stay out of the picture and let us find a way of eating that is enjoyable and is right for each individual. Perhaps we all can't lose weight by following the same rules. <u>Maybe we need to change the rules.</u>

It is now December 2014 and I have been changing the way I eat since the end of August. I have lost a total of 30 pounds, with many more to go. But I am not discouraged because the changes I have made in my diet have not been hard to follow. They are not big changes. They have not been painful changes. In fact, the new way I have been eating has made me have fewer cravings and leaves me satisfied and the satisfaction stays with me longer. (Has the diet industry been steering us wrong on what a proper diet is?)

Follow me as I continue my journey and see if the things that I learned about eating and dieting will work for you, because "IT WORKS FOR ME."

CHAPTER 1

Giving Up Sweets

"Giving up sweets"

As I pondered just what I could do to lose weight, I decided to go low carbs. I have known people who have lost weight this way and it seems to work. By carbs, I mean sugar and starches. Many have tried this diet and do ok for awhile but then fail. Why is it so hard to stick to? Why do they fail? If I take this low carb diet and tweak it to my own needs, make it something that I can stick with, and then I can follow this formula and maybe I will see the results that I want.

Carbohydrates are sugar and starches which our bodies need to function well and they provide us with energy. Some carbs are healthier than others.

First, let us look at sugar. Sugar is the simplest of carbs. It occurs naturally in some foods including fruits (fructose), milk and milk products (lactose) and table sugar (sucrose). The table sugar is the one that I avoid whenever possible. Table sugar is what I am referring to when I say I gave up sugar. This includes things made from table sugar - baked goods, coffee cakes, donuts, etc. It also includes things like jellies and candy, foods with 10 grams or more of sugar added. I just use my own judgment. If it tastes sweet – forget it.

Most low carb diets have strict rules. No sugar and no bread, noodles, white rice, white pasta, cereal, and no white potatoes. Nothing made from white flour. Makes me wonder what I can eat. Some diets say not to eat anything white. I know that I can't stick to this way of eating for long.

So I decided to create my own diet with my own rules. I needed to be able to live with this diet so I kept it simple.

Rule #1: No sugar

Rule #2: No bread (meaning bread, bagels, English muffins and rolls)

It is easy to remember and nothing to count or measure. If it resembles sweets or bread, I do not eat it. I could do this. Just give up two things. That's all just two things. I tried it and guess what, it worked. I began seeing results my first week.

My fear was that giving up sweets was going to be difficult. I eat sweets several times a week. I have done this for as long as I can remember. I had to have something sweet after the evening meal, even if it was only a bite or two of cake or a piece of candy.

When eating at a restaurant, the waitress always asks if I want dessert. Well, of course I did, even if I was full. When gathering with my siblings, there is always plenty of food and more than enough desserts. How was I going to resist temptation?

Well I knew it was necessary and also possible. Sugar is not a diet food!

It was not as hard as I thought it would be. After only a few days, my desire for sweets went away. What made me desire these sweets in the first place? The more I ate, the more I wanted. I needed to break this cycle. I stopped eating sweets "cold turkey." It is the best way to end this addiction. It didn't take long before I lost my desire for sweets. Sugar is now the last thing I crave. Tables full of sugary goodies are no longer tempting to me.

When I was a baby, my mom fed me every four hours. If I cried between feedings and appeared hungry she would give me a bottle of water with some syrup or sugar added. In those days many mothers sweetened water for their babies. Since it tasted better to her I guess she thought it tasted better to me.

Do babies really have a preference? Are they able to tell if something tastes sweet or sour? In the 1940's it was thought that a baby needed to drink water. So my mother, being the good mother that she was, would make my water taste better according to her taste.

I not only had sugar in my water, but as soon as I was a few weeks old I was given rice baby cereal. Mom tasted the cereal and it tasted so bland that she would spice it up with (you guessed it), a spoonful of sugar. This was surely the beginning of my addiction to sugar. Today's mothers feed an infant on demand

and doctors say that it is not necessary for them to have water. Times have changed.

My need for sugar only grew from there. As a child, I remember my mom spending hours in the kitchen baking. There were cookies, cupcakes, pies, donuts, sweet rolls and at times even fudge. She made the best chocolate cake with chocolate peanut butter frosting. Our house would smell so good when she was in the kitchen baking and the best part was eating warm sweets fresh out of the oven.

We always had something sweet in our school lunches. I used to wish that just once I could have a store bought cookie or cupcake in my lunch like the other kids. I didn't realize how lucky I was to have such a wonderful mother who loved to bake.

In a pinch when there were no sweets in the house, we would eat sugar sandwiches (yes, you heard me right, a sugar sandwich). This delicious treat consisted of two pieces of white enriched bread, smothered with a lot of real butter and in between the two slices of bread was a quarter inch thick layer of brown sugar.

Another substitute for baked goods was a layer of frosting between two graham crackers.

These sweets that I ate as a child, prepared by a loving mother, would send the food police scurrying today.

There were times our entire evening meal was nothing but sweets! When she baked apple dumplings, we would eat them warm, fresh from the oven, swimming in milk. That would be our entire dinner. On Sunday after church, we would always have chicken for our noon meal and for our evening meal we would just have ice cream, that's all, just ice cream, each and every Sunday. I even remember on occasion for breakfast having left over elderberry pie drowning in milk. Even a healthy dish of fruit, like a dish of sliced up peaches or strawberries was sprinkled with sugar.

Despite the large amounts of sugar my siblings and I ate as children, we were not overweight. I don't know why. Was it because we got more exercise than kids today? Was it because our food was fresh and homemade without preservatives? Maybe the reason was that it was real sugar, not the artificial kind (sugar substitute). I'm not sure. What I do know is that we had a wonderful SWEET childhood.

As great as this sounds and with all the love and caring in which the sweets were given, it helped form my need for sweets. This was my comfort food. A comfort food being a food that is psychologically comforting, especially food that is high in carbohydrates. It is a food that when we eat it as an adult we enjoy very much and often eat when we need comfort. So maybe this is why I grabbed a candy bar when I was bored or depressed.

I know there must be more to the need for sweets than just giving us comfort. Before I started this journey, the more sweets I ate the more sweets I wanted. What causes this? Is there a chemical reason? Why did the cravings stop when I stopped eating sweets?

Eating sugar can be addictive. It can be a family tradition that brings comfort and also it can become a habit. Eating sweets can make you happy and avoiding them can make you crabby. Whatever it does chemically to my brain, I'm not sure. But I know that the more I have the more I want. Even when I try to avoid it, it sneaks into my life. This battle for me has ended. Am I saying, I will never eat sweets again, of course not? I allow myself a treat on special occasions and to be sociable, but I can do without sweets just fine.

Health wise, sweets increase your waist size, increase your risk for Type 2 diabetes, elevate your triglyceride and increase your risk for heart disease. Diets high in sugar are linked to depression, migraines, poor eye sight, autoimmune disease, gout and osteoporosis. No matter how much I researched the only good thing that I found about sugar is that it tastes so good.

In the 1960's the first diet soda came out. I didn't care for it much. It left a bad aftertaste in my mouth. Eventually the artificial sugars improved in taste and they began to be more widely used in many processed foods. Are these sweeteners good for us? They contained no calories; this seems like a good thing. Were there also some Bad Things about this no calorie sugar?

Some experts say artificial sugars have the same effect on your body as sugar and therefore keep you from losing weight. (If artificial sugar has the same effect on our bodies as sugar, what is the point of using them?) I don't use these substitutes. Who invented this sweetener? Why didn't scientists know the effects of this substance on our bodies? I believe that they may be harmful.

The American obesity epidemic has been occurring simultaneously with the increased use of artificial sweeteners. They also increase the yearning for more sweets and may disrupt normal metabolism. We trust the Food and Drug administration to ensure everything we eat is healthy. How healthy are these sweeteners? We put our trust in experts, doctors, and the FDA to help us with our struggles with weight control. But can we trust them? I'm not sure and that is why I decided to make my own rules for eating healthy and my own rules for losing weight.

As far as drinking diet soda or regular soda, I don't drink them. I have come to the conclusion that water is the best no calorie beverage. Water also reduces hunger, helps hydrate your skin and keeps your body working efficiently. What a great drink. Do we need these nasty chemicals from substitute sugars in our bodies? Perhaps we stayed thin as kids because we ate natural foods not chemicals.

You would think with my family history of excessive sweets it would be difficult for me to give up sugar. I was surprised that it was relatively easy. With sweets out of the picture, I also lost the desire to snack.

I also don't read labels too much in regards to the amount of sugar in a food. I keep this diet simple; if it tastes sweet, I don't eat it. Surprisingly I am no longer the least bit interested in eating sweets. They can be right in front of me and I am not tempted. I do not deny myself a treat on a few occasions, but very rarely, and then only a small serving.

Since I removed sugar from my diet, my energy level stays high. I don't have the ups and downs that I once experienced. I am so glad that I kicked my addiction to sweets. And it wasn't that hard to do, if I can live without sweets, with a history like mine, so can you.

CHAPTER 2

Giving Up Breads

"Giving up breads"

Bread is the second thing that I gave up on my diet journey. By bread, I mean English muffins, bagels, and rolls as well as bread. This was a little more difficult than the sugar. I love bread and was used to eating it, sometimes at all three meals, each and every day. I would have toast or a bagel or an English muffin for breakfast, most always a sandwich for lunch, and many times a roll or garlic bread with my evening meal. That's a lot of bread.

Bread is a starch. To stop eating starches completely is not a good idea. Starches are an important part of a healthy, balanced diet. Starches are made of many sugars bonded together. They appear naturally in vegetables, grains, dry beans and peas. Starches need to be chosen correctly and consumed in the right portions. White enriched bread is not one of the correct choices!

Fiber is a special type of carbohydrate that passes through the digestive system virtually unchanged. Fiber makes food more filling; it lowers blood sugar, lowers cholesterol and may even prevent colon cancer. It is found naturally in fruit, vegetables, whole grains, dry beans and peas.

As I began this diet, I wondered what I could eat if I did not eat bread. What would I have with my coffee in the morning? What would I eat for lunch if not a sandwich? It's strange what you think you cannot live without.

After a short time following my new diet plan, I realized that I could be just as satisfied by substituting the white bread with better choices. Eggs and bacon with a side of fruit is now one of my favorite breakfast meals.

Another good breakfast is a bowl of whole grain cereal topped with nuts and fruit swimming in milk. It fills me up and keeps me satisfied for hours. I know what you are thinking, "Cereal on a low carb diet." Well, this is Low carbs not No carbs.

We all know whole grains are good for us. I am careful of the cereal I choose. I do not eat sugar coated cereal and only those made of whole grains. I also pay attention to the portion size. The way to stick to this new way of eating is to eat and enjoy food without feeling deprived. I still sometimes think about having a sandwich at lunchtime, but I discovered that I am just as satisfied with meat and cheese with vegetables and mayonnaise, wrapped in a whole wheat tortilla.

Some experts say white potatoes should be avoided when you are dieting to lose weight. Too much starch they say. I believe potatoes are an excellent source of potassium which is important to maintain a healthy blood pressure and the skin of a potato is a good source of fiber. What is so bad about that? I love white potatoes. I did not give up eating white potatoes and I still lost weight!

Beans are one of the healthiest options. They are a good source of fiber. They are a plant based protein and are packed with nutrients and antioxidants.

The starches that should be avoided are not the whole grains. Whole grains are good because of their ability to lower cholesterol. The ones that have been refined, meaning the nutrients and fiber rich parts are removed and processed; are not good for you. According to the American Diabetes Association, the best way to identify healthy grain is to check the ingredient list. Make sure the first ingredient in starchy food is whole wheat flour, brown rice, rye flour, barley or oats.

I wanted this diet to be simple and didn't want to read labels so I avoided any and all bread. Maybe when my weight is stabilized I will introduce the right kind of whole grain bread into my diet.

Like sweets, my love for bread began early in my life. Growing up, I ate toast for breakfast, sandwiches for lunch and there was always bread on the table for our evening meal. We didn't have just any bread; it was often the Italian or French bread that comes long, uncut and still warm from the grocery store bakery. It would be wrapped in white paper, and with a wonderful aroma. Applying real butter and having it melt into the bread was pure heaven.

A short time after giving up bread, I began to realize that I no longer had cravings for potato chips, popcorn, pretzels or other salty snacks. I began to wonder if eating sweets and/or bread was making me hungry and unsatisfied after a meal. The more carbohydrates, I ate the more I seemed to want and the more weight I would gain.

Eating bread causes your blood sugar to go up. When your blood sugar goes up rapidly it tends to go down rapidly. When your blood sugar goes down, you feel hungry. People on high carbohydrate diets eat, eat, eat. Soon after eating, they become hungry again and reach for another high carbohydrate snack. Before you know what has happened, you have gained some extra pounds and can't seem to get off this cycle. This describes how I was eating and this is why many people can't lose weight. They continue to eat the wrong kind of carbohydrates and therefore are soon hungry again.

When I say that I gave up bread, I am not talking about a diet that is free of starchy carbohydrates. White bread is made of refined flour and contains little nutritional value.

I allow myself whole grain cereal a few times a week. I eat white potatoes; I'm not sure why low carb diets exclude them. I eat pizza and white pasta occasionally, although I try to eat smaller portions than I used to and eat a salad to fill me up. If I eat rice, I try to eat brown rice; I like it as well as white.

By eating all these foods I love in reasonable size servings and omitting bread, I am able to go between meals without snacking. I am satisfied and do not feel the need to snack. Three meals a day, no bread and no sugary sweets and I am on my way to my dream weight.

By not eating bread, just like sugar, my craving for it has disappeared.

I started this diet by just giving up these two things, bread and sugar. My weight started coming off at the rate of a pound or two a week. This has been so simple. I don't feel deprived, I don't feel hungry and I am taking off those unwanted pounds, slowly but surely.

My doctor has recently checked my cholesterol and the ratio between the good and bad cholesterol has improved. He said to keep doing what I am doing because IT WORKS FOR ME.

CHAPTER 3

Adding More Fats

"Adding more fat"

As I continue on this path of diet modification, I wonder what else I can change to improve my health through my diet. How about adding fat to my diet? Yes, I said adding fat. I know this shocks most people.

Is it possible that the "experts" have been promoting diet "myths" that were wrong? I think so because my food choices don't match most of their recommendations and yet I am losing weight every week or two. There are some weight loss rules that I am throwing out the window.

Like I said before, I am not an expert; I have no degree in nutrition. Something just does not add up when we try to lose weight doing what these experts tell us and instead the weight continues to climb.

I know that this sounds a bit crazy, but again I think the experts who tell us what we should and should not be eating are wrong. Since the 1970's and 80's we have been told that "eating a fatty diet will make us fat and clog our arteries." So the grocery stores started filling their shelves and coolers with low fat and no fat foods. There were low fat versions of just about every kind of food. Everyone started buying low fat food. Well, like everyone else, I too bought these foods hoping to lose weight, only to find out that the weight continued to climb.

The average weight of Americans began to

increase with the introduction of sugar substitutes and low fat foods. Heart disease is on the rise and there are now more people on statin drugs than ever before. Don't these experts see this is not working?

Saturated fat is a perfectly natural part of the human diet. Is it possible that there has been faulty research about saturated fat? Have the so called experts been wrong for the last five decades?

In Finland the selling of low fat and no fat food is banned. Only 13% of their population is obese. In the U.S. 33% of the population is obese. They also have less heart disease than the U.S. and less people on statin drugs.

Several tribes in Africa have diets that consist of mostly raw whole milk, lots of red meat and cow's blood. They eat five times the saturated fat that we do in the United States and yet they have lower heart disease, body fat and less people with diabetes. (I have to say that I draw the line at drinking cow's blood.)

Certain Pacific Island nations eat food very high in total fat and yet they are very lean and have no heart disease. When these islanders moved to the U.S. and ate less saturated fat and more processed food, they started developing heart disease.

The Mediterranean culture has one of the healthiest diets in the world. They eat fruit, vegetables, whole grains, nuts and olive oil. They get 35-40% of their nutrients from fat. These people eat a higher percentage of fat in their diets and yet have much lower heart disease than the rest of the world.

We are told by the experts that we should decrease our LDL (bad cholesterol); to do that they say that we should limit our fat intake. We should avoid saturated fat. We should eat low fat foods and no fat foods. Have you tasted no fat food? "Yuck" is all I have to say.

Saturated fat intake increases LDL (bad cholesterol), and increases HDL (good cholesterol). This improves your overall cholesterol ratio. Your cholesterol ratio is more important than your total cholesterol.

Another thing I want you to think about here is trans fat or trans fat acids. This type of unsaturated fat is uncommon in nature, but can be created artificially. Many foods in our country are fried using this man made vegetable oil. "Vegetable" oil sounds healthy, but don't be fooled. This is the worst kind of fat. The vegetable oil industry has taken over oil for cooking. French fries, fish, chicken, appetizers are fried in this unhealthy oil. Before this oil was created, lard or butter was used for frying. The country was not fat then.

If you become a label reader, avoid foods that include "partially hydrogenated oils" on the list of ingredients; they are the Trans fats. Hydrogenated or partially hydrogenated oil should be avoided and eliminated from your diet. If a label lists "partially hydrogenated oil," don't buy it!

The vegetable oil industry is a billion dollar business and so is the cholesterol medication industry. Neither one is about health; it's all about profit. Makes you wonder doesn't it?

Now another oil that has been around since the 1970's is Canola Oil. Is Canola Oil good or bad for us? Friends and family have been saying it is the healthiest oil out there. I've been hearing a lot about this oil lately, so I decided to Google it on the web.

Canola Oil is produced from a seed of varieties of the rape plant, namely of rapeseed or field mustard. It is genetically modified refined oil. The word canola comes from "Canada Oil" and is not a naturally grown plant. I bet you never knew that.

The rapeseed is toxic to human and other animals. Rape seed is the number one ingredient of toxic pesticides. Now that's a scary fact! Anything that is produced from a plant that is also an ingredient in a pesticide is not going in my body! "They" insist that through genetic engineering it is no longer rapeseed but canola. According to the Canola Council of Canada, it is considered safe for human consumption. There are many claims of unhealthy side effects from

Canola Oil. No long term research has been done to substantiate or refutes the claim.

The Canadian government paid our Federal Food and Drug Administration $50 million dollars to have Canola Oil placed on the GRAS list (Generally Recognized as Safe).

I didn't realize how powerful and influential the food oil industry is until I started researching Canola Oil. Stop and think about it – the oil industry controls every processed food we eat at home and every meal we eat at restaurants, especially fast food restaurants. Their profits are huge – billions of dollars a year! I think it's safe to assume that profit is their main goal, not the health of their consumers. They "pretend" to be health conscious. They advertise promoting Canola Oil as a healthy choice, but in my opinion, it is not.

This oil is found in many processed foods - margarine, peanut butter, breads, and most potato chips. After doing this research, I think I must now become a label reader. Again, I have to say I do not always believe the experts when it comes to my health. I prefer virgin olive oil, grape seed oil or butter for cooking.

Ignoring the experts I have added fat to my diet. I do not mean that I eat food that is fried in oil. I don't eat French Fries or deep fried meat or appetizers.

24

I Do Eat bacon and cheese and real butter, I know that is shocking, but I am still losing weight!

When a food is labeled "low fat" or "fat free," often sugar is added to maintain flavor. Sugar is the main reason I believe I gained so much weight.

Looking at all these facts made me want to try something different in my effort to lose these extra pounds I have been carrying around for a long time. I decided to start putting more fat in my diet. I no longer eat "lite" and "no fat" foods. I eat animal fat and dairy fat and I have to say that it took some courage to get over the fear of fat that was drummed into my head for so long. I no longer believe that eating fat makes us fat or that it increases our cholesterol levels and causes arteries to clog. The fat in food enhances the taste and is much more satisfying. I believe that by removing fat from our diet we are harming our bodies and therefore our health.

I eat eggs (which the so called experts at one time said were bad for us, now they say that they are ok). I eat cheese, 4% cottage cheese, milk and even bacon. Although I haven't switched to whole milk yet, I did go from drinking skim to drinking 2%. (It may take awhile for me to make the switch from eating low fat foods that I ate for over 40 years).

I have found that eating fat makes me feel satisfied and that satisfied feeling lasts longer.

Therefore, I do no snacking between meals and often do not feel hungry at meal time. By eating food that contains dairy and animal fat, I am eating less food and I don't feel deprived at all.

A Swedish doctor, Andreas Eenfeldt, said that fat is the best thing for losing weight and maybe the most effective. Could this be true?

Is this low fat, no fat food the answer? I now believe fat has been falsely labeled "bad" by the experts. Look at the facts. Americans on average are fatter and have higher cholesterol levels since this "eating fat makes you fat" thing started. This DOES NOT WORK FOR ME.

There are other factors that also contribute to health and weight. What have the "experts" said about exercise and proteins in our diets? Are they also wrong about their advice in these two areas?

Chapter 4

Protein and Exercise

"Protein and Exercise"

I believe proteins are needed for energy. They build and repair tissue. They are needed to make enzymes, hormones and other body chemicals. Unlike fat and carbohydrates, the body does not store protein and has no reservoir to draw on when it needs a new supply. Proteins are found in meat, poultry, fish, legumes, tofu, eggs, milk and milk products, nuts, seeds, grains and some vegetable and fruits. When protein intake is inadequate, the body cannibalizes protein from muscles and organs.

Proteins perform many different functions to sustain your life. About 10 to 30% of your daily calorie intake should come from protein. Protein contains about 4 calories per gram, and can serve as an energy source when needed. Proteins are important to every cell in the body. Hair and nails are mostly made of protein.

Some recommended protein sources are fish, poultry, beans, nuts and whole grains. Plant-based food like soy and legumes contain the same amount of protein as meats and nuts. Nuts not only give you a lot of protein, but they are a healthy source of fat. You need not worry if you are eating a well balanced diet, because you are probably getting enough protein. Healthy people rarely need protein supplements.

I make sure that I eat enough protein in a day so that I have energy to keep going. Since I have added more protein to my diet, my metabolism has increased and, therefore, more fat is burned.

I put nuts on my cereal and salads. I eat meat and fish. I eat eggs and cheese and cottage cheese. Natural peanut butter is a great source of protein; I like it occasionally on celery.

I think by eating protein throughout the day my energy level is maintained. I don't have the highs and lows that I once had when I was eating sugar and breads. A good diet is about balance. Cut back on foods high in simple carbohydrates and stock up on veggies, fruits, complex carbohydrates and lean protein. Fats, proteins and carbohydrates are all equally important parts of our diets.

In regards to exercise, I have to say that I do not agree with the "experts" again. I do not believe that "calories in, equals calories out." Experts say that obesity is just a matter of eating too many calories and that the only way to reduce your weight is to eat less and move more. This way of thinking just does not make sense to me. Does it not matter where you get your calories? All food does not have the same reaction in our bodies. The experts say that, if you eat less calories than you burn you will lose weight and, if you eat more calories than you burn, you will gain weight. Focusing on the calorie content of a food and disregarding the metabolic affects they have on the body is why, in my opinion, people are not losing weight. Can 300 calories of sugar have the same affects on the body as 300 calories of protein? The answer is no. You cannot out exercise a bad diet!

Forget calorie counting; eat a healthy diet of fats, protein and plenty of low glycemic carbohydrates, such as fruits and vegetables and exercise moderately.

I'm not against exercise. It is good for your bones, muscles, lungs, heart and overall wellness. I just don't think that exercising to burn calories you take in will result in a permanent weight loss, because all calories are not created equal.

Children today seem to play much differently than we baby boomers did. We were very active, spending much of our day outside. We would run, jump rope, and ride our bikes. We played hopscotch and tag. The winter cold did not keep us inside. We were outside sledding, making igloos, making snowmen and forts, and having snow ball fights.

My whole family once built a snowman as big as the house. We named him big Tex (he had bowed legs). We were getting exercise and breathing in that fresh cold winter air and creating the best memories. It was great exercise for the entire family.

Winter fun is not what it used to be. In the

past, you would drive down a street and see children building snowmen or igloos in every yard. I don't see that any more. Do children even have snow ball fights in this modern world? I saw in the stores not long ago a toy being sold that surprised me. It was a snowman building kit. It included a hat, button eyes, a scarf and buttons for the coat. It even included a plastic carrot for a nose. You mean to tell me kids can't find these things for themselves. Half the fun in building a snowman is running around and finding the things to decorate him. Hat and scarves were always around the house and mom would have a real carrot waiting for us. We would dig in the snow for stones to use as eyes, mouth, and buttons.

Roller skating and ice skating are great exercise, are these popular anymore?

Today's children are not active. They are often in front of the TV or on their computers. They play games using their fingers. Where is the exercise that they need to grow? What happened to running and playing hide and seek or flashlight tag?

I see elaborate swing sets in back yards of beautiful homes, but very seldom see any children swinging. Is having a nice swing set in your yard just a status symbol now? I remember when I was young swinging for hours trying to reach the sky. My swing set was not elaborate or fancy. My dad made it out of pipes, chains and it had wood seats. He painted it red. It remained in my parent's back yard for decades.

Even as teenagers we were very active. Marching in the high school band, dancing, bike riding, roller skating. We were involved in a lot of activities and busy with our friends.

We were active as a family too. We were campers and spent many wonderful hours in nature. What happened to that easy and active way of life?

Adults don't get the exercise like they used to either. Exercise is essential for our health. There are too many modern conveniences today. I am thinking about the way my mom spent one entire day a week washing clothes for our large family. She went down the basement steps with the laundry. Using a wringer washer, she would wash the clothes (wring the clothes), rinse the clothes (wring the clothes). Carry the heavy, wet clothes up the steps, into the back yard and hang them on a clothes line. She would bend, stretch, pin – bend, stretch and pin for every piece of clothing we had worn all week. That is an exercise none of us has to do today, thankfully. Not to mention stretching, unpinning and folding each piece, and carrying them into the house. She didn't have to go to the gym to exercise. She got plenty of exercise just doing the laundry.

In today's world we put the laundry in the

washer, push a button and go read a book. No exercise in that. It's the same thing when we wash dishes. Just put them in and push a button. We don't have much need to iron anymore, nor do we do much cooking from scratch. The time that we now spend on daily chores takes much less energy.

The work my dad did was much more physical than a great deal of jobs today. After working at a shop as a pipefitter, he would come home and work in the garden or fix things around the house. There was no repair man called to work on our cars or to do any of the home repairs. It was all done by dad.

Because of the way they worked and lived and played 50 years ago they did not need to set time aside to exercise. The way they lived they didn't need to exercise.

Because times have changed, we do need to set aside time to exercise in order to stay healthy. We do not move enough to keep us strong. How much exercise is enough? I don't think we need to train for a marathon. We need to spend time doing more physical things. We need to spend more time in nature. Just taking a daily walk or going on a bike ride is all that is needed to improve our health. Gardening is another great exercise. Anything that will get us moving will nurture our bodies and our minds.

CHAPTER 5

Today's Diets

Today's diets

Today's diets are quite different than those of 50 or 60 years ago. What has become of the diets of the past? The experts that we listened to for too long have made us afraid of fats, eggs, red meats and many other healthy foods.

Many years ago American grew most of their own food. Women, would can the food or freeze it so the family could enjoy fresh fruits and vegetables year round.

Today much of our food is processed and then delivered to the grocery store. During the processing, ingredients are added, such as sweeteners (or artificial sweeteners), preservatives and stabilizers. This process changes the nutritional value of a food. Have you ever read the labels on processed food? If I don't recognize the ingredients or can't pronounce them, then I don't buy it.

I recently bought a loaf of bread and put it in my pantry. I left it there for three weeks and it still was not moldy. What had been added to the white enriched wheat to allow it to last for so long? During the holidays I saw a billboard sign that read "fruit cakes have a shelf life of 25 years." Really? That's a bit too many preservatives for me.

In the early 1950's, the TV stared to become a standard for most American homes. Along with the

TV came one of the first processed meals, the TV dinner. It included a full meal with a dessert. For many this became an easy and fast meal, just heat it in the oven and eat.

Then came the microwave in the 70's. Ready to eat meals became the norm. More women were working and wanted easy to fix meals for their families. The processed food industry grew from there. The processed food could be easily prepared and served, but was it good for us?

Processing food affects the nutritional value of a food. It transforms the food physically or chemically. Certain additives can result in an addiction to a particular food. The pathway that food takes between the place of origin and your plate should not be through a processing plant. I try to avoid food that has been ultra processed like those labeled "ready to eat."

Recently I have been hearing more about "clean eating." This is eating whole foods or real food, foods that have been minimally processed, and as close to their natural form as possible, foods that have been unprocessed or minimally processed. This way of eating can be challenging these days. Clean eating excludes foods with additives of any kind and foods that have been manufactured in labs.

Some processed food is not so bad because the processing removes toxins and bacteria (i.e., milk) It is not bad to freeze or can in season fruits and vegetables. Some minimally processed foods such as unrefined grains, frozen fruits and vegetables also are not bad. Clean eating does not mean eating everything raw. It means eating minimally processed food with few ingredients added. Ultra processed food should be avoided.

Some people who follow the so called clean eating diet also eat organic food. I do not eat organic, but often look at the food labels to see where the food originated. After all, can we believe that a food is really organic just because it says on the label?

Recently a method called "cleansing" has become popular in the health world. The purpose of cleansing is to detox your body and rid it of unhealthy toxins by flushing them out with liquid fruits and vegetables. It has become a 55 million dollar business and growing. The cleansing requires making a juice of fruits and vegetables. Many go on juice cleansing for 3-5 days or up to a couple of weeks. The promise is that your hair will shine and your skin will shimmer, you will have tons of energy and it will clear your mind and you will lose weight. However, juice cleansing is not a good way to lose weight.

By liquefying fruits and vegetables you eliminate the fiber which aids in digestion. This can't be good. You shed water weight, but it comes back when you start eating.

This is another of those ideas that make others very rich while harming our bodies. Our body is very unique and is able cleanse itself. The liver and kidney are our body's detoxification system. They continually remove waste products and toxins.

Eating out is a scary thing to me. Looking at the menu and trying to decide the healthiest option is sometimes difficult. Many of the choices are fried or have such names as chicken fingers (chicken have fingers?) or fish sticks (?), or a basket of chicken wings (where's the rest of the chicken?).

I believe a big contributor to the obesity epidemic in this country is the amount of fried food that is consumed and the frequency of dinning out by the average American. When I was young and SKINNY, my family only ate out a few times a year.

Everything is fried in today's world, vegetables (onions, cauliflower, mushrooms, pickles, potatoes,) fish, chicken, shrimp. Since I no longer include fried food in my diet, I have a hard time finding a healthy choice when I eat out. Most meals are served with a side of fries. Some restaurants can even ruin a salad by topping it with fried chicken strips.

Recently when I was attending the county fair, I walked past a food stand selling deep fried Twinkies and deep fried Oreos. That is an example of a bad food choice made worse! When I think about the amount of fried food that is consumed, it's easy to see how we became an obese nation.

Not only what you eat, but the amount you eat matters. Servings are larger than they have ever been. It used to be that when you ordered a hamburger and fries you got a small hamburger on a small bun with a small order of fries. Now most people want a double or triple hamburger with a layer of bun between each meat patty. The french fries went from a small order to a large order to a super size order.

When eating the wrong kinds of food, you're hungry faster and you end up wanting more. When you are eating the right food, you are satisfied with less.

There are many factors that determine the amount of food our bodies need. Are you a marathon runner or a person with a sedentary job? It also depends on a person's age and health. Each of us needs to tweak our diets to meet our own needs.

Weight gain happens for many reasons. Sometimes we eat after we are full, we eat because we're bored, and we eat when we're not hungry. We skip meals and then snack late at night. Eating at a certain time of day is something I have always done. We need to eat based on hunger, not the clock. We need to listen to our bodies in order to maintain a healthy weight.

Over the years, we have been given conflicting diet information. How do you know what is right for you? I do not think there is a diet that is a "one size fits all" solution to weight loss. I believe it is trial and error. Each person needs to find what works for him or herself.

As a country we have seen many diets come and go – low fat, no fats, low carbs, dairy free, gluten free, eggs being a cholesterol nightmare, sugar free, sugar substitutes, no red meats and the list goes on and on.

Smoking, excessive drinking of alcohol and obesity all disrupt our bodies. To be healthy, we need to stop abusive behaviors, exercise more, play more and eat right.

I believe that we need to "be in the moment." By this, I mean when you are out for a walk "be in the moment." Look around you, smell the flowers, see the animals and insects around you. Think only of what is around you at that moment in time. Listen to your footsteps and your breathing. Feel the breeze or sun on your face. Observe nature. Push your troubles away for a short time while you are on your walk.

This "in the moment" practice should also be applied when you are eating. Smell your food, chew your food slowly, feel the texture on your tongue. Do not eat while in front of the TV, this is mindless eating. Do not eat while reading a book or newspaper. Listen to your body when it tells you that your stomach is full and then stop eating even if it still tastes great. While you are eating "be in the moment."

CHAPTER 6

This Is What Works For Me

"This is what works for me"

The word "diet" means what a person usually eats and drinks. When most people think of the word "diet" they connect it with a deprivation or a punishment. They think a diet is something that is hard to do and is sometimes painful, in truth it does not have to be. Try thinking of it as a positive life change not the dreadful and boring denial of eating foods that you love.

In 1863 William Banting wrote a pamphlet – "Letter on Corpulence" which he wrote to the public. He is known for being the first to popularize a weight loss diet based on limiting intake of refined and easily digestible carbohydrates. His diet plan consisted of four meals a day: Protein, Greens, Fruit and Dry Wine. Avoid Starch and Sugars. Milk, butter and meat were all permitted. AVOID STARCH AND SUGAR. That is exactly what I have been saying. He was about my age when he began this way of eating and lost (like I am) a pound a week. A diet of long ago and it is still working today; there must be something to it.

My goal the first week on this diet was just to try something different; a way of eating that was satisfying and easy. No calorie counting and no points assigned to foods. No measuring and deprivation of foods. It sounded like an impossible mission.

I anxiously started that first day by getting on

the scale and facing the reality of my actual weight. I pulled out a sheet of paper and wrote down the date and the large number that the scale showed. This was my beginning weight. I always use the same scale and have on the same amount of clothing, or in my case, my so called birthday suit. I always weigh myself the first thing in the morning before I eat or drink anything. Every Saturday morning I get on the scale and record my weight beside the date.

Where do I start? I decided to start with the carbohydrates that I eat in excess. I didn't want to be too strict with this new journey. Not cutting out all carbs, I love white pasta and pizza. I wanted a diet that I could stick to. I removed sugary foods and bread (including English muffins, bagels, rolls and anything else that looked or smelled like bread). That's it, sugar and bread. This I could do.

When week one was over, I reluctantly approached the scale. Thinking that I did not reduce my food intake by very much, I was not expecting any weight loss. There was the number. I was down one pound. Wow! Ok, on to week two, three, four and five. Yep it works, five weeks and down 5 pounds. This may not seem like much weight, but I was not hungry or deprived and it was in the right direction. And I was very happy losing one pound a week because I know that it is not healthy to lose a lot of weight at once.

After several more weeks, the weight continued to disappear a pound a week. I continued with no sugar or bread. I began to add more protein to my diet and my energy soared. I recently removed low fat food from my diet and continue to lose.

One week I stayed the same weight and at Christmas time I had a week with a two pound gain, only to have a 4 pound loss the following week. Every other week I had at least a one pound loss. It has now been over 5 months and my total weight loss is 41 pounds!

I recently had my doctor check my cholesterol and it showed an improved cholesterol ratio. The foods I eat are not low fat or low calorie. My average day goes something like this.

For breakfast, I like whole grain cereal with fruit and nuts, or an egg fixed like an omelet folded over with cheese in the middle. Sometimes I add two slices of bacon. Remember, no bread and no sugar. Don't be afraid of fat and add protein to your meals. I usually have a piece of seasonal fruit each morning. This keeps me satisfied for at least 5 hours with a lot of energy.

Lunch usually consists of a salad with lettuce, veggies, nuts, fruit, cheese, leftover meat from the night before or anything else I can find to put in it, followed by a piece of fruit. There are times I really crave a sandwich, so then I take some meat and cheese and veggies and wrap them in a whole wheat tortilla spread with a little mayonnaise (not the low fat kind). And I add a piece of fruit. This keeps me satisfied until the evening meal.

Dinner is meat, potatoes, veggies and a salad or cottage cheese. Occasionally I have two slices of pizza and a salad. Pasta is something I love and I eat it once in awhile with a salad. This satisfies me until morning.

I find by eating this way I no longer have the desire to snack or eat between meals and I do not get hungry. I do not feel that I deprive myself of anything. The amount of food that I eat is less than I ate prior to starting this new way of eating. I believe eating sugar and bread made me feel the need to eat more and I would get hungry in a short time.

Like I said before, I am no expert and a lot of people will say that I am eating the wrong foods. After all, how many diets have you been on that allow bacon, red meat, allows you to eat until you are full and bans fat free food?

Eating out when I was dieting always was a challenge. Not now. Salad is a good choice or any food as long as it's not sweet and it is not bread or fried in oil.

I have not at this point started an exercise routine. I do think it is an important part of a healthy life style. I love hiking a wooded trail and enjoy bike riding on the rail trails. Walking is an exercise that can be done anywhere and is my exercise of choice. I think that moderate exercise is all that is needed for healthy bones, joints, muscles and overall wellness.

Diet pop, with artificial sugar and regular pop, with sugar, are not allowed. I prefer hot green tea and water for my beverages. I try to drink a lot of water and keep it by my side and sip it throughout the day.

As the weight started to come off, week after week, I was even more committed to this new way of eating. It felt so easy compared to the rigid diets that failed in the past. I do not look at this way of eating as a weight loss diet, but as a change in my eating habits. The weight loss is just a side benefit.

Sometimes on special occasions, such as a birthday celebration or a holiday, I have found myself surrounded with tasty sugary desserts. I tell myself it is ok to enjoy the treat. I take a small portion and truly savor it without guilt.

No calorie counting, no measuring, no points assigned to food. Just eat what you like and watch the weight come off.

As we age, we know that it is harder to lose weight. I am 68 years old and have tried for many years to lose weight, but finally I found a "diet" that "WORKS FOR ME."

If you have decided to follow my Revolutionary Way of Eating, I wish you luck in your weight loss, and hope you discover that it will "Work For You" too!

SANDY'S EASY DO'S AND DON'TS

DON'T EAT	DO EAT
Sugar	Everything Else
Artificial sugar	
Bread	
(Bagels, muffins, rolls)	
Soda	
(Diet or regular)	
Low fat foods	
No fat foods	
Vegetable and canola oil	

www.ingramcontent.com/pod-product-compliance
Lightning Source LLC
Chambersburg PA
CBHW071126280526
45787CB00003B/1191